E.A. VICTORIA

HOW TO BECOME THE GIRL OF YOUR DREAMS

*A female's guide to leveling up in health, finance, &
Relationship*

First edition

This book was professionally typeset on Reedsy.
Find out more at reedsy.com

To the woman who shaped my world with love, wisdom, and grace—my mother. Though you're no longer by my side, your spirit continues to guide and inspire me every day. In loving memory of the extraordinary woman you were, this book is dedicated to you. Forever in my heart.

Contents

1

Introduction

Have you ever found yourself scrolling through social media, just flipping through feeds or posts of those girls who seem to have it all? The beautiful house, an amazing lifestyle, cute-looking pets, and sometimes a very attractive partner who adores them. They always appear to have enough money to travel, look fashionable, or just seem to be having so much fun and living their best lives.

And then there's you. Maybe you've just returned from your long 9-to-5 job where the pay isn't great, but you have bills to pay, so you just suck it up and work for the money (there's absolutely nothing wrong with working for your money). Or maybe your case is a bit different. Perhaps you're a stay-at-home mom or partner, or a single mom with kids. Whatever the case, you look around, and the life you are currently living is not really what you had in mind for yourself.

Well, not to worry. This short book is my love letter to you. Think of me as your fairy godmother, your big sister, your girly girl, or bestie. I am here to help you transform your life from where you are currently to where you want to be. Maybe you just want enough money to quit your day job and travel the world without a care in the world. Or maybe you are more concerned with getting that high-value partner, man, or woman, the person that just adores you, sweeps you off your feet, showers you with love and gifts (if that is your love language). Whatever your case may be, no matter how old you are, through this book, we are going to become THE girl, the girl of your dreams.

In this book, we are going to tackle the big three. I like to call them the big three because I believe they are the foundation on which becoming your dream girl stands. The big three being health, finance, and relationships. Over the course of this book, I am going to guide you on how to fix these three. If any one of them is not where it is supposed to be, once you have the big three in order, I am sure you can become the girl of your dreams.

Please note, this is a short book to guide you; it goes in-depth into some topics and not so much into others. I wanted the book to be easy to read. You can always use it as a reference or guide on your journey to becoming the girl. Also, if you identify as male, non-binary, or something else, everyone is welcome. You can also use this book as a guide in your leveling up journey.

So to my beautiful girlie girls, princesses, and queens, it's time to put on your crown and get to work. Your guide is here to guide you to become THE girl, so consider this a workout session. Let's get to work.

2

PART ONE: HEALTH

Hey there, bestie, welcome to the first session of "Becoming the Girl of your Dreams." The first thing we are going to tackle is our health because, as the saying goes, health is wealth. We can't be girl of our dreams if our health isn't in order. Also, what good would it be if you had all the money in the world and not the good health to enjoy it?

So, whether you are a big girly who wants to lose weight in a healthy way or you are a queen who wants to watch what she eats and make sure she is eating healthy because, as they say, you become what you consume, or maybe your case is a bit different. Maybe you want to lose some stones and go down a few pounds to get your ideal body type. Don't worry, big sis has got you all. I have got some health tips and workout lists for all kinds of ladies, from my pregnant girlies to my girlies with limited mobility.

Healthy food to help lose weight
I won't be listing specific foods you have to eat, because depending on the region of the world you reside, some of these food items might not be available, but in order to eat healthy, here are some foods you need to

incorporate into your diet.

Vegetables: Rich in fibre, vitamins, and minerals, vegetables are low in calories and high in nutrients. Include a variety of colourful vegetables such as leafy greens, broccoli, carrots, and bell peppers in your meals.

Fruits: Fruits provide natural sweetness along with fibre and essential vitamins. Opt for whole fruits rather than fruit juices to benefit from the fibre content. Berries, apples, and grapefruit are good choices.

Lean Proteins: Protein is crucial for weight loss as it helps maintain muscle mass and keeps you feeling full. Include sources of lean protein such as chicken breast, turkey, fish, tofu, legumes, and low-fat dairy products.

Whole Grains: Choose whole grains over refined grains for added fiber and nutrients. Quinoa, brown rice, oats, and whole wheat products are excellent choices.

Healthy Fats: Include sources of healthy fats in moderation, such as avocados, nuts, seeds, and olive oil. These fats provide satiety and support overall health.

Legumes: Beans, lentils, and chickpeas are rich in fiber and protein, making them great choices for weight loss. They also have a low glycemic index, which helps stabilize blood sugar levels.

Greek Yogurt: Greek yogurt is higher in protein and lower in sugar compared to regular yogurt. It can be a satisfying and nutritious snack or breakfast option.

Water: While not a food, staying well-hydrated is essential for overall health and can contribute to weight loss by helping control appetite. Drink water throughout the day, especially before meals.

Green Tea: Some studies suggest that the catechins in green tea may help with weight loss by boosting metabolism and promoting fat burning. It also provides a low-calorie beverage option.

Spices and Herbs: Flavor your meals with herbs and spices instead of relying on high-calorie sauces and dressings. Many herbs and spices have additional health benefits and can add variety to your meals.

Natural food with health benefits

I have also handpicked some specific food items, which I believe are great and have several health benefits.

Berries: Blueberries, strawberries, raspberries, and blackberries are rich in antioxidants, vitamins, and fiber. They may help improve cognitive function and protect against oxidative stress.

Leafy Greens: Spinach, kale, Swiss chard, and other leafy greens are packed with vitamins (such as A, C, and K), minerals, and fiber. They contribute to overall health and may help reduce the risk of chronic diseases.

Nuts and Seeds: Almonds, walnuts, chia seeds, and flaxseeds are sources of healthy fats, protein, and fiber. They can help reduce inflammation and support heart health.

Fatty Fish: Salmon, mackerel, and sardines are rich in omega-3 fatty acids, which are beneficial for heart health, brain function, and reducing inflammation.

Turmeric: Curcumin, the active compound in turmeric, has anti-inflammatory and antioxidant properties. It may help with conditions such as arthritis and may have potential anti-cancer effects.

Garlic: Garlic has anti-bacterial and anti-viral properties and may help lower cholesterol levels and support heart health.

Honey: Honey offers various health benefits, including antioxidant properties, wound healing, and soothing a sore throat. It contains natural sugars, enzymes, and trace amounts of vitamins and minerals.

Avocado: Avocado is a nutrient-dense fruit rich in healthy monoun-saturated fats, vitamins, and minerals. It supports heart health and may aid in weight management.

The foods listed above would absolutely help you lose weight, but you also have to remember, it's essential to focus on overall dietary patterns rather than specific foods alone. Portion control, moderation, and a balanced approach to nutrition are key components of a sustainable and healthy weight loss journey. Additionally, consulting with a healthcare professional or a registered dietitian can provide personalized guidance based on your individual needs and health status.

Substance abuse and self-control

In the spirit of discussing what we put in our bodies, I want to use this opportunity to talk about substance abuse and self-control.

In order for you to become the girl, you have to have extreme self-control and discipline. You cannot become the girl you want to be without forgoing momentary pleasure and bad habits. One of the biggest bad habits you have to break, if you are currently in that situation, is substance abuse—be it drugs, alcohol, excessive caffeine, smoking, or vaping. One of the biggest problems with the substances listed above is that they are extremely addictive, and once your brain gets used to them, it is usually very difficult to break the habit.

This means you become a slave to this substance; your brain craves it, and this could be a distraction in your journey to becoming the girl. Instead of focusing on how to achieve something or make your next move, your brain would be working extra hard on getting the substance it is addicted to. This can lead you down a dark path, resulting in financial issues (spending all your money getting high), homelessness, or finding yourself in difficult situations—all because you got your brain addicted to the wrong thing.

Not to worry, if you have some habits you are trying to break, I have provided some tips you can use to break some of these destructive habits.

Tips on how to break destructive habit

Awareness and Acknowledgment:

· Recognize and admit that the habit is destructive.

· Understand the negative impact it has on your life and well-being.

Set Clear Goals:

· Define specific, measurable, achievable, relevant, and time-bound (SMART) goals for breaking the habit.
· Break down larger goals into smaller, manageable steps.

Understand Triggers:

· Identify situations, emotions, or environments that trigger the habit.
· Develop strategies to cope with or avoid these triggers.

Replace with Positive Habits:

· Replace the destructive habit with a healthier alternative.
· Focus on building positive habits that align with your goals.

Seek Support:

· Share your goal with friends, family, or a support group.
· Surround yourself with people who encourage and support your efforts.

Professional Help:

· Consider seeking guidance from a therapist or counselor.
· Professionals can provide strategies and tools to address underlying issues.

Mindfulness and Meditation:

· Practice mindfulness to increase awareness of your thoughts and actions.
· Meditation can help you develop greater control over impulses.

Positive Reinforcement:

· Celebrate small victories along the way.
· Reward yourself for achieving milestones in breaking the habit.

Visual Cues:

· Use visual reminders to stay focused on your goal.
· Create a vision board or set up reminders on your phone.

Learn from Setbacks:

· If you slip up, don't be too hard on yourself.
· Analyze what led to the setback and use it as a learning opportunity.

Develop Coping Strategies:

· Build healthy coping mechanisms for stress or challenging situations.
· Exercise, deep breathing, or engaging in hobbies can be effective.

Track Progress:

· Keep a journal to track your progress.
· Document challenges, successes, and how you feel throughout the

process.

Make Environmental Changes:

· Modify your environment to reduce the likelihood of engaging in the habit.
· Remove items associated with the habit from your surroundings.

Remember, breaking a habit takes time and persistence. Be patient with yourself and stay committed to the positive changes you're making. If needed, seek professional assistance for additional support.

Mental Health

You absolutely cannot become your dream girl, if your mental health is not in order, so it is important that you mind, and body are in alignment. There are different types of mental health issue, and we won't be able to cover all in this book, but here are some tips on how to get your mental health in order.

Tips on how to get your mental health in order

Seek Professional Help:

· If you're struggling with mental health issues, consider reaching out to a mental health professional. Therapy and counselling can provide valuable support and strategies for managing challenges.

Establish a Routine:

· Create a daily routine that includes regular sleep patterns, healthy meals, and consistent exercise. A structured routine can provide stability and contribute to mental well-being.

Exercise Regularly:

- Physical activity has a positive impact on mental health. Aim for at least 30 minutes of moderate exercise most days of the week. This can include activities like walking, jogging, or yoga.

Prioritize Sleep:

- Ensure you get enough quality sleep each night. Lack of sleep can negatively impact your mood, concentration, and overall mental health.

Practice Mindfulness and Meditation:

- Incorporate mindfulness and meditation practices into your routine. These techniques can help reduce stress, improve focus, and enhance your overall mental well-being.

Connect with Others:

- Foster social connections with friends, family, or support groups. Spending time with others can provide emotional support and combat feelings of loneliness.

Limit Screen Time:

- Set boundaries on your screen time, especially on social media. Excessive use of digital devices can contribute to stress and negatively impact mental health.

Healthy Nutrition:

- Maintain a balanced and nutritious diet. Nutrient-rich foods can positively impact your mood and energy levels.

Limit Alcohol and Substance Use:

- Be mindful of alcohol and substance use. Excessive consumption can negatively affect mental health. If you're struggling, seek professional help.

Set Realistic Goals:

- Set achievable and realistic goals for yourself. Break larger tasks into smaller, manageable steps to avoid feeling overwhelmed.

Learn to Say No:

- Prioritize your mental health by learning to say no when needed. Avoid overcommitting yourself and recognize your own limits.

Cultivate Hobbies:

- Engage in activities you enjoy and that bring you a sense of fulfilment. Hobbies can provide a healthy outlet for stress and contribute to a positive mindset.

Challenge Negative Thoughts:

- Practice cognitive-behavioural techniques to challenge negative thoughts. Replace negative self-talk with more positive and realistic perspectives.

Take Breaks:

- Schedule breaks throughout the day to rest and recharge. Avoid burnout by giving yourself time to relax and step away from work or stressful situations.

Regular Check-ins:

- Regularly check in with yourself. Pay attention to your emotions and feelings and be proactive in addressing any concerns.

Remember that mental health is a dynamic and individualized aspect of well-being. It's okay to seek professional help and make adjustments to your lifestyle to prioritize your mental health. If you're struggling, don't hesitate to reach out to a mental health professional or talk to someone you trust.

<u>workout routines</u>

After prioritizing healthy eating and ensuring that what we put inside our bodies positively impacts our health, let's shift our focus to the physical aspect. We not only want to feel good but also look healthy. I understand that everyone's metabolism is different, and what works for one person might not necessarily work for another. Therefore, I've created a variety of workout routines tailored for girls of various sizes and abilities.

If you find that you can't do any or all of the workout routines listed below, that's perfectly fine. The important thing is to find something that works for you and your body type. The most crucial aspect is to keep working on yourself. As Martin Luther King Jr. said, "If you can't fly, then run. If you can't run, then walk. If you can't walk, then crawl. But whatever you do, you have to keep moving forward."

Consistency is key, so aim to make physical activity a regular part of your daily routine. Remember, progress is progress, no matter how small, and taking steps towards a healthier you is a significant achievement.

Simple daily workout routines

Warm-up (5 minutes):

· Jumping jacks or jumping rope to elevate your heart rate.
· Arm circles, leg swings, and gentle stretches for flexibility.

Cardiovascular Exercise (15-20 minutes):

Choose one or a combination of activities:

· Brisk walking or jogging in place.
· Cycling, either outdoors or on a stationary bike.
· Dancing to your favourite music.
· High-intensity interval training (HIIT) with activities like jumping jacks, burpees, or mountain climbers.

Strength Training (15 minutes):

Bodyweight exercises are effective:

· Squats: 2 sets of 15 repetitions.
· Push-ups: 2 sets of 10-12 repetitions.
· Lunges: 2 sets of 12 repetitions per leg.
· Plank: 2 sets, holding for 30 seconds to 1 minute.

- Flexibility and Mobility (10 minutes):

Stretching exercises to improve flexibility:

- Neck stretches.
- Shoulder stretches.
- Hamstring stretches.
- Chest opener stretches.
- Yoga poses like Downward Dog or Child's Pose.

Cool Down (5 minutes):

- Light jogging in place or walking to gradually lower your heart rate.
- Deep breathing exercises.
- Gentle full-body stretches, holding each stretch for 15-30 seconds.

Remember to listen to your body, and if you have any existing health concerns or conditions, consult with a healthcare professional or fitness expert before starting a new exercise routine. Additionally, feel free to modify the routine based on your preferences and gradually increase intensity or duration as your fitness level improves.

Simple daily workout routine for pregnant ladies

Bestie, exercise during pregnancy can be beneficial for your overall health and well-being, but it's crucial to consult with your healthcare provider before starting or continuing any exercise routine. Assuming you have received clearance from your healthcare professional, here's a simple daily workout routine for my pregnant ladies. Make sure to adapt it based on your comfort level, and listen to your body throughout:

Warm-up (5 minutes):
·Gentle marching in place.
·Arm circles and shoulder rolls.
·Pelvic tilts to engage your core.

Cardiovascular Exercise (15-20 minutes):
·Brisk walking is a safe and effective option.
·Swimming or water aerobics can be gentle on joints.
·Low-impact aerobics or modified dance workouts.
·Strength Training (10-15 minutes):

Bodyweight exercises can be beneficial:
·Squats: 2 sets of 12-15 repetitions.
·Standing leg lifts: 2 sets of 12 repetitions per leg.
·Seated rows with resistance bands: 2 sets of 12-15 repetitions.
·Modified push-ups against a wall or on an incline: 2 sets of 10-12 repetitions.

Prenatal Yoga or Stretching (10 minutes):
·Gentle yoga poses designed for pregnant women.
·Pelvic tilts, cat-cow stretches, and hip openers.
·Stretching for the back, legs, and shoulders.

Pelvic Floor Exercises (5 minutes):
·Kegel exercises to strengthen pelvic floor muscles.
·Pelvic tilts to engage and release the pelvic muscles.

Cool Down and Relaxation (5 minutes):
·Slow walking or marching in place to bring your heart rate down.
·Deep breathing exercises or guided relaxation.
·Gentle stretches for the entire body.

Tips for Safe Exercise During Pregnancy:

·Stay hydrated and avoid overheating.

·Wear comfortable clothing and supportive shoes.

·Avoid exercises that involve lying flat on your back after the first trimester.

·Modify or skip exercises that cause discomfort or pain.

·Listen to your body and take breaks as needed.

·Focus on maintaining good posture throughout your exercises.

Workout Routine for my girlies with limited mobility

Warm-up (5 minutes):

·Seated March: Sit on a stable chair and lift one knee at a time in a marching motion.

·Arm Circles: Slowly rotate your arms in small circles, gradually increasing the size.

Cardiovascular Exercise (10-15 minutes):

·Seated Marching: Continue with seated marching, increasing the pace slightly for a cardiovascular effect.

·Seated Leg Taps: Extend one leg forward, tapping the floor, and then switch to the other leg.

Strength Training (10 minutes):

·Seated Leg Lifts: Lift one leg at a time, holding briefly before lowering.

·Seated March with Resistance: Use resistance bands around your legs while seated and perform marching movements.

·Seated Bicep Curls: Hold light weights or use resistance bands for seated bicep curls.

Flexibility and Mobility (10 minutes):

·Seated Neck Stretches: Gently tilt your head from side to side, forward, and backward.

·Seated Shoulder Rolls: Roll your shoulders forward and backward to ease tension.

·Seated Hip Stretch: Cross one ankle over the opposite knee and gently press down on the crossed knee.

Balance Exercises (5 minutes):

·Seated March with Alternating Arm Raises: Lift one arm at a time while marching in place.

·Seated Leg Extensions: Extend one leg forward and hold briefly for balance.

Cool Down and Relaxation (5 minutes):

·Seated Forward Bend: Gently reach forward while sitting to stretch the back.

·Deep Breathing: Inhale deeply through the nose, exhale through the mouth, focusing on relaxation.

·Seated Cat-Cow Stretch: Round your back and then arch it, alternating between the two positions.

Remember to move within your comfort zone, and if any exercise causes pain or discomfort, stop immediately. Adjust the intensity, duration, and type of exercises based on individual abilities and limitations. It's always a good idea to seek guidance from a physical therapist or fitness professional.

These are just a few workout routines you can follow for your body type and workout needs. If any of these workouts don't meet your needs, you can always search online for one that's best for your unique needs. Now that we have, or are getting, our health and body in order, the next thing we have to do on our path to becoming THE GIRL is to get our finances in order because your dream girl has her finances in order.

3

PART TWO: FINANCE

Hi beautiful ladies, welcome to the second pillar of becoming your dream girl. In this session, we would be talking about finances, so let's get right to it. Unless your mom or dad is rich (and even that is risky), you absolutely cannot depend on anyone for your financial stability. I cannot stress this enough; as a lady, being financially independent is extremely important. There is a golden rule that says, "He who owns the Gold makes the Rule".

As the girl, there is no way we would be depending on someone for our finances, and I'm sure some of you might be saying, "Oh, I will just marry a rich man, and that would solve my financial problem." Ladies, I don't know how to put this lightly, so let's do some girl math using the United States as an example because it is the country with the most millionaires. Let's say you are a young girl in your 20s and you want to marry a rich guy or girl who is a millionaire. Well, out of the around 20 million people living in the USA that are millionaires, only 1% of millionaires are below the age of 35, so around 200,000 males and females. Currently, we have 43 million girls between the ages of 20 – 40. As you can see, the competition for that 1% would be huge.

There just aren't enough rich young people to go around. You would probably have to share him/her with someone else. Besides, placing all your financial plans on someone else might just not work in your favor, especially if you live in a country where the justice system isn't that strong. You might end up divorced in your 30s, 40s, or even 50s, with nothing on your resume and no financial support. I could write for hours about why it is extremely risky to base your finances on someone else, but I won't go that far because my smart girlies know it is plain dumb to put all your eggs in one basket.

In this session, I would be discussing how you can level up financially no matter your current situation – single mom, recent grad, stay-at-home mom, matured ladies who just want to be financially free. I'm going to be discussing money, how to make it, how to save it, and how to grow it so you can one day quit your 9-to-5 job.

Education, Car, & Career

Education

To my beautiful sisters, I am here to tell you that education still remains the key. I'm sure you have heard the saying, "Oh, getting a degree is not important. You can still make it without a degree. Education is a big money scam," etc.

Well, if you do a bit of research, you would find out that the odds of you making it big without an education are very low. The higher your education, the better. Studies have shown that people with bachelor's degrees make significantly more than people with high school diplomas, and people with master's degrees, on average, make more than those with just a bachelor's. So yes, education does, in fact, help you become financially independent.

Below, I have listed a few reasons why I think everyone should get educated.

Advantages of getting an Education

Increased Job Opportunities: Education opens a wider range of career options and increases your chances of finding employment. Many professions require a certain level of education as a basic qualification.

Higher Earning Potential: On average, individuals with higher levels of education tend to earn more over their lifetimes. Education can lead to better-paying jobs and increased earning potential.

Personal Development: Education contributes to personal growth and development. It enhances critical thinking, problem-solving skills, and the ability to make informed decisions.

Improved Health and Well-being: Studies have shown a positive correlation between education and health outcomes. Education equips individuals with the knowledge to make healthier lifestyle choices and access better healthcare.

Enhanced Social Skills: Through education, individuals develop social skills, communication abilities, and teamwork, which are essential for success in personal and professional relationships.

Civic Engagement: Education fosters civic responsibility and community involvement. Educated individuals are more likely to participate in civic activities, vote, and contribute to societal development.

Critical Thinking and Analytical Skills: Education cultivates critical thinking skills, enabling individuals to analyze information, make reasoned judgments, and approach challenges with a problem-solving mindset.

Personal Fulfilment and Confidence: Acquiring knowledge and skills through education can lead to a sense of personal achievement and fulfillment. Education builds confidence and a sense of empowerment.

Adaptability and Lifelong Learning: Education equips individuals with the ability to adapt to new situations and learn continuously. Lifelong learning becomes a natural part of an educated person's journey.

Social Mobility: Education is a powerful tool for social mobility, allowing individuals to move beyond their socioeconomic backgrounds and achieve upward mobility.

Global Perspective: Education broadens one's perspective, fosters cultural understanding, and prepares individuals to engage in a globalized world.

Personal and Financial Independence: Education often contributes to personal and financial independence. It provides the skills and knowledge needed to navigate the challenges of life and make informed financial decisions.

Well, I hope with these few points, I have been able to convince you as to why you need to get educated. I'm sure some of you have questions regarding getting educated—questions like, how do I fund my studies without going into debt? Or, I think I'm too old to get educated, or I don't have time to go back to school; I have a family to run, etc. Yes, these are all valid reasons that might stop you from getting educated. What we would not do in this journey is make excuses. It's easy to make excuses, but what we would do is find solutions.

Thanks to the internet, you can pretty much get many free resources to help you build the skill set you need. Below, I have listed some ways to fund your studies. Also, for my girls just getting started or still trying to figure out what to study, I always say, do your research. If you are trying to become financially free as quickly as possible, you should consider going for programs where people get paid well. Science, Technology, Engineering, and Maths (STEM) are usually well-paid. I'm sure you might say, "But I don't like math." I understand. Following your passion is a good thing, but sometimes you have to go where the money is, else you won't be able to afford to follow your passion

If following your passion can pay the bills, then by all means, go for it. But if you want to enjoy your passion without worrying about money, you have to consider going for high-paying jobs. It mustn't be STEM programs; finance, economics, etc., also pay. All I'm trying to say is make sure to major in something you can rely on to get a good paying job.

Currently, there is a huge pay gap between men and women; on average, men make more money, and also, we have more men in STEM programs than women. Maybe there is a correlation between these two; maybe more girls need to occupy more STEM spaces. We need to break the glass ceilings and occupy spaces. I want to see more female scientists, astronauts, pilots, civil, structural, computer, electrical, chemical engineers, etc. Alright, back to funding our education.

How to Fund your Education

Scholarships and Grants:

- Research and apply for scholarships and grants. Many organizations, institutions, and foundations offer financial aid based on academic achievement, extracurricular activities, and other criteria.

Federal Student Aid (FAFSA):

- Complete the Free Application for Federal Student Aid (FAFSA). This form determines your eligibility for federal grants, loans, and work-study programs. It's an essential step in accessing federal financial aid.

Work-Study Programs:

- Explore work-study opportunities on campus or within your community. These programs allow you to work part-time to earn money for educational expenses while gaining valuable work experience.

Part-Time Employment:

· Consider part-time work during the school year or full-time employment during breaks to help cover living expenses and tuition costs.

Internships and Co-op Programs:

· Look for paid internships or co-op programs related to your field of study. Some employers may provide financial assistance or even cover tuition costs for students participating in these programs.

529 Savings Plans:

· If your family has set up a 529 savings plan, it can be used to cover qualified education expenses, including tuition, books, and room and board.

Community College or In-State Schools:

· Consider starting at a community college or attending an in-state public university to reduce tuition costs. Many community colleges have transfer agreements with four-year institutions.

Online Courses and Programs:

· Explore online courses or programs, which may offer flexibility in scheduling and can sometimes be more cost-effective than traditional on-campus programs.

Private Loans:

- If needed, consider private student loans. Be cautious with private loans, as they often have higher interest rates than federal loans and fewer repayment options.

Crowdfunding:

- Use crowdfunding platforms to raise funds for tuition and related expenses. Share your story and goals, and reach out to friends, family, and your community for support.

Military Service:

- Consider joining the military, as many branches offer educational benefits, such as the GI Bill.

Employer Tuition Assistance:

- If you're working, check if your employer offers tuition assistance or reimbursement programs for employees pursuing higher education.

Here are a few ways you can fund your studies. The most important thing is acquiring the required marketable skill sets to help you secure a well-paying job, so you can start making some real money, get your finances in order, and become THE GIRL.

Note: Getting an education is obviously not the only way to make money. Other methods will be discussed in this book, but having a higher education certainly makes it a lot easier. So, if you can, do get it.

Car

To become the girl, you might actually need a car, especially if you live in a country like the USA, which has so much landmass, and everything is spread out. If you live in a country with a good public transport system, you might be able to do without a car. However, if you need a car, then you have to find ways to get one because it literally gives you your freedom.

With a car, you are free to go wherever you want; it's your car. Perhaps you've just started your new job, and you need a car to get to work. Maybe you need to run some errands – you need a car. Now, how do you finance your car? Also, take note; it mustn't be a really expensive or super flashy car. If that's what you want and can afford it, go for it. But for my girls who are just starting and need a reliable car to get them from point A to point B, here are a few tips on how to finance.

Usually, I would advocate that you get a reliable used car if you are just starting off, and then later, when you have the means, you can upgrade. But to each his own.

Smart ways to finance a car

Improve Your Credit Score:

· A higher credit score often leads to better loan terms and lower interest rates. Before financing a car, work on improving your credit by paying bills on time and reducing outstanding debt.

Save for a Down Payment:

· Saving for a substantial down payment can lower the amount you need to finance and decrease your monthly payments. Aim for at least 10-20% of the car's purchase price.

Compare Loan Offers:

- Shop around for financing options. Check with different lenders, including banks, credit unions, and online lenders, to find the most favorable interest rates and terms.

Understand Loan Terms:

- Read and understand the terms of the loan, including the interest rate, loan duration, and any additional fees. Be aware of the total cost of the loan over its life.

Consider Pre-Approval:

- Get pre-approved for a car loan before visiting dealerships. This allows you to know your budget and negotiate from a position of strength.

Negotiate the Price:

- Negotiate the price of the car separately from the financing terms. Dealerships may offer better financing rates if they know you're a serious buyer.

Avoid Extended Warranties and Add-Ons:

- Be cautious with extended warranties and additional add-ons offered by dealerships. They can significantly increase the total cost of the loan.

Choose the Right Loan Term:

- While longer loan terms may result in lower monthly payments, they can also lead to higher overall interest costs. Choose a loan term that aligns with your budget and financial goals.

Refinance if Necessary:

- If your credit improves or interest rates drop after you've secured the initial loan, consider refinancing to get a better rate.

Budget for Additional Costs:

- Factor in additional costs such as insurance, maintenance, and fuel when budgeting for your car. This ensures you can comfortably manage all associated expenses.

Consider Used Cars:

- Buying a used car can be a cost-effective option. Used cars typically depreciate more slowly than new cars, and they often come with lower insurance costs.

Pay Attention to Total Cost of Ownership:

- Consider the total cost of ownership, including insurance, maintenance, and fuel efficiency. A more fuel-efficient and reliable car can save you money in the long run.

Remember to thoroughly research and understand the terms and conditions of any financing arrangement before committing. If possible, seek advice from financial experts or consult with a trusted financial advisor.

Career

I know some might enjoy it, while others may hate it and wish they never have to go to work. I hear you, girlies; I know sometimes it can get boring. The truth is, unless you have super-rich parents who can give you money to start your dream business or you have a supportive spouse who can afford to pay you to be a stay-at-home partner, the truth is we all need to make that money, and having a job is one way of making money. The secret is not staying there longer than you have to. So, you have that degree, a skill you use to make money, your car; now is the time to grind. Now is the time to make the money which we would use to gain our financial freedom. Here are some tips on how to have a fulfilling career.

Tips on how to have a fulfilling career

Self-Reflection:

- Take time to reflect on your skills, strengths, passions, and values. Consider what truly matters to you in a career and what gives you a sense of purpose.

Set Clear Goals:

- Establish both short-term and long-term career goals. Define what success looks like for you and the steps you need to take to achieve those goals.

Explore Your Interests:

- Explore different industries, job roles, and career paths. Networking, informational interviews, and internships can provide valuable insights into various fields.

Continuous Learning:

· Stay committed to learning and professional development. Acquiring new skills can make you more adaptable and open up new opportunities for career growth.

Networking:

· Build a professional network by connecting with colleagues, mentors, and industry professionals. Networking can provide valuable guidance, support, and potential job opportunities.

Work-Life Balance:

· Prioritize work-life balance to avoid burnout and maintain overall well-being. A healthy balance allows you to perform better in your job and enjoy your personal life.

Seek Feedback:

· Be open to feedback from colleagues, supervisors, and mentors. Constructive feedback can help you identify areas for improvement and growth.

Embrace Challenges:

· Don't shy away from challenges. Embrace them as opportunities for learning and growth. Overcoming obstacles can lead to a greater sense of accomplishment.

Build Strong Relationships:

- Cultivate positive relationships with colleagues, superiors, and subordinates. A supportive and collaborative work environment contributes to career satisfaction.

Express Your Ideas:

- Share your ideas, innovations, and perspectives with your team or organization. Contributing to discussions and projects can make you feel more engaged and valued.

Stay Flexible:

- Be adaptable to changes in the workplace and industry. A flexible mindset allows you to navigate uncertainties and seize new opportunities.

Align Values with Employer:

- Choose employers whose values align with yours. Working for a company that shares your values can enhance your sense of purpose and satisfaction.

Pursue Passion Projects:

- If possible, incorporate aspects of your passions into your work. This can bring a sense of fulfillment and purpose to your career.

Evaluate and Adjust:

- Periodically evaluate your career satisfaction and progress. If necessary, be willing to make adjustments, whether it's changing roles, industries, or pursuing additional education.

Remember that a fulfilling career is a journey, and it's okay to reassess and make changes along the way. Regularly check in with yourself to ensure that your work aligns with your values and brings you a sense of fulfillment.

Debts and building credit

We have our money-making career, our 9 am to 5 pm job, or our business that generates income during the day. Now is the time to pay off our debts and build up our credit. To do this, it takes discipline because lifestyle inflation can be a big problem. At this point, you have to stay focused. The only way you are going to become THE GIRL is to become financially free, and you need money-generating assets to do that. The only way you are going to get money-generating assets is by using money. In other words, you need to use money to make money.

Back to the topic of lifestyle inflation, you can be making six figures and still be living paycheck to paycheck. This is where good money management and budgeting habits come into play. Below are some good money management habits you can adopt to help you retain what you get paid.

Good Money Management Habit

Budgeting:

· Create a realistic budget that outlines your income, expenses, and savings goals. Track your spending regularly and adjust your budget as needed.

Emergency Fund:

- Establish and maintain an emergency fund to cover unexpected expenses. Aim to save three to six months' worth of living expenses in a readily accessible account.

Savings Goals:

- Set specific savings goals for short-term and long-term needs, such as an emergency fund, vacations, or a down payment for a home. Automate your savings to make it a consistent habit.

Live Below Your Means:

- Avoid overspending and strive to live below your means. Differentiate between needs and wants, and prioritize essential expenses while cutting back on unnecessary purchases.

Avoid High-Interest Debt:

- Minimize the use of high-interest debt, such as credit cards with outstanding balances. If you have debt, work on paying it off as quickly as possible.

Credit Score Monitoring:

- Regularly check and monitor your credit score. A good credit score is essential for obtaining favourable interest rates on loans and credit cards.

Investing for the Future:

- Start investing for the long term. Take advantage of employer-sponsored retirement plans, such as 401(k)s, and consider additional investment options, like IRAs or taxable brokerage accounts.

Review and Adjust:

- Periodically review your financial situation and goals. Adjust your budget, savings, and investment strategies as your circumstances change.

Insurance Coverage:

- Ensure you have adequate insurance coverage, including health, life, and property insurance. Insurance protects you and your family from unexpected financial setbacks.

Smart Shopping:

- Be a conscious consumer. Look for discounts, compare prices, and avoid impulsive purchases. Consider buying in bulk and taking advantage of sales and promotions.

Educate Yourself:

- Continuously educate yourself about personal finance. Stay informed about investment options, tax strategies, and other financial matters that impact your money management decisions.

Negotiate and Shop Smart:

- Negotiate when applicable, whether it's for a salary, service, or a big purchase. Additionally, shop around for better deals on insurance, utilities, and other recurring expenses.

Retirement Planning:

- Plan for retirement early. Contribute consistently to retirement accounts and take advantage of employer matches if available.

Regularly Assess Financial Goals:

- Reassess your financial goals periodically. Adjust your goals based on changing life circumstances, such as marriage, having children, or changes in employment.

Mindful Spending:

- Practice mindful spending by consciously evaluating your purchases. Consider the value and impact of each expense on your overall financial goals.

Consistency is key when it comes to money management. By developing these habits and integrating them into your daily life, you can build a solid foundation for financial success and security.

How to build your credit score

A good credit score is crucial for various financial activities such as loan approval, good interest rate, renting a house, credit card approval and terms, security deposit, employment opportunities. Below are some tips on how to build a good credit score.

Check Your Credit Report:

- Obtain a copy of your credit report from each of the three major credit bureaus (Equifax, Experian, and TransUnion) at least once a year. Review the reports for any errors or discrepancies.

Establish a Credit History:

· If you don't have a credit history, consider applying for a secured credit card. Secured cards require a security deposit but can help you build credit. Make small, regular purchases and pay off the balance in full each month.

Become an Authorized User:

· Ask a family member or friend if you can be added as an authorized user on their credit card account. This can help you build credit by having the account's positive history reflect on your credit report.

Apply for a Starter Credit Card:

· Look for credit cards designed for individuals with limited or no credit history. These cards may have higher interest rates, but they can be a useful tool for building credit when used responsibly.

Pay Your Bills on Time:

· Consistently pay all of your bills on time. Timely payments have a significant impact on your credit score. Set up reminders or automatic payments to avoid late payments.

Keep Credit Card Balances Low:

· Aim to keep your credit card balances low relative to your credit limit. High credit utilization can negatively affect your credit score. Ideally, keep your credit utilization below 10%.

Diversify Your Credit Mix:

· Having a mix of different types of credit accounts, such as credit cards, installment loans, and retail accounts, can positively impact your credit score. However, don't open new accounts just for the sake of diversity.

Limit New Credit Applications:

· Avoid applying for multiple credit cards or loans within a short period. Each application can result in a hard inquiry, which may temporarily lower your credit score.

Pay Off Debts:

· Work on paying off existing debts. Reducing outstanding balances can positively impact your credit score over time.

Negotiate with Creditors:

· If you're struggling with debt, consider negotiating with creditors for more favorable terms. Some creditors may be willing to work with you on a repayment plan.

Seek Professional Advice:

· If you're facing significant credit challenges, consider seeking advice from a credit counselor. Non-profit credit counseling agencies can provide guidance on managing debt and improving your credit.

Be Patient and Consistent:

- Building credit takes time. Be patient and consistent in your efforts to make positive financial decisions. Over time, your credit history will reflect responsible behaviour.

Remember that building credit is a gradual process, and it's essential to maintain good financial habits over the long term. Regularly monitoring your credit reports and scores can help you track your progress and identify areas for improvement. Following the tips listed above would definitely put you on the track to getting you fincece is order. The next part is how to grow our wealth.

Side hustle, Business, and investments

Great job, Queens! You're making money and building up your credit. Now, it's time to grow your wealth because, let's be real, the goal is financial freedom. The aim is to let your money work for you, giving you free time to enjoy the things you love, rather than constantly working for money.

In this section, I'll discuss some side hustles you can work on while keeping your full-time job to make extra cash. If your side hustle becomes significant enough to cover your bills, you can consider working on it full-time. But until then, keep your day job. We don't quit our day job without a game plan.

Some side hustle you can do, while keeping your 9 to 5 Job
Freelancing:

- Offer your skills as a freelancer in areas such as writing, graphic design, web development, social media management, or marketing

Online Tutoring or Coaching:

- Share your expertise by offering tutoring or coaching services online. This could include academic subjects, language learning, or professional skills.

Consulting:

- If you have industry-specific knowledge, consider offering consulting services to businesses or individuals.

Virtual Assistance:

- Provide virtual assistance services to businesses or entrepreneurs, helping with tasks such as email management, scheduling, and administrative support.

E-commerce:

- Start an online store on platforms like Etsy or Shopify, selling handmade crafts, vintage items, or print-on-demand products.

Photography:

- If you have photography skills, consider offering services for events, portraits, or stock photography.

Real Estate:

- Get involved in real estate by becoming a part-time real estate agent, property manager, or real estate investor.

Fitness Coaching:

- If you're passionate about fitness, become a part-time fitness coach or instructor, either in person or online.

Blogging or Content Creation:

- Start a blog or YouTube channel focused on your interests or expertise. Monetize through advertising, sponsorships, or affiliate marketing.

App or Web Development:

- If you have programming skills, take on freelance projects for app or web development.

Stock Market Investing:

- Learn about stock market investing and consider investing a portion of your savings. Keep in mind that investing involves risks, so it's important to do thorough research.

Event Planning:

- Offer event planning services for weddings, parties, or corporate events on weekends or during your free time.

Social Media Management:

- Provide social media management services to businesses or individuals looking to improve their online presence.

Survey Taking or Market Research:

- Participate in online surveys or market research studies during your free time to earn extra income.

Language Translation:

- If you are fluent in multiple languages, offer translation services for documents, websites, or communication materials.

Before starting any side gig, ensure that it aligns with your skills, interests, and available time. Additionally, be mindful of any potential conflicts of interest with your full-time job and consider consulting your employer or reviewing company policies if necessary. Always prioritize a healthy work-life balance to avoid burnout because we are trying to become THE GIRL, not burnout princesses. Health above wealth.

Now we have money, here are some places you can invest your money to let your money work for you.

<u>Investment Options</u>

Stock Market:

- Invest in individual stocks or exchange-traded funds (ETFs) based on thorough research and a well-defined investment strategy.

Real Estate:

- Invest in rental properties or real estate investment trusts (REITs) for potential long-term returns.

Cryptocurrency:

- Consider investing in cryptocurrencies like Bitcoin or Ethereum but be aware of the associated risks and volatility.

Retirement Accounts:

- Contribute to retirement accounts such as a 401(k) or IRA for long-term wealth accumulation.

Peer-to-Peer Lending:

- Explore peer-to-peer lending platforms where you can lend money to individuals or small businesses for returns.

Dividend Stocks:

- Invest in dividend-paying stocks to receive regular income from your investments.

Mutual Funds:

- Diversify your investment portfolio by investing in mutual funds managed by professional fund managers.

Start-ups and Small Businesses:

- Consider investing in start-ups or small businesses that align with your interests and expertise.

Precious Metals:

· Invest in precious metals like gold and silver, which can act as a hedge against economic uncertainty.

Education and Skills Development:

· Invest in your education and skills development to enhance your career prospects and income potential.

Before starting a business or making investments, it's crucial to conduct thorough research, seek professional advice if needed, and carefully assess your risk tolerance. Diversification and a long-term perspective are often key elements of a successful investment strategy.

We have our health in order, we are working on our finances, and we have all the tips to gain financial freedom. Now, let's talk about the last pillar to becoming your dream girl.

4

PART THREE: RELATIONSHIPS

<u>We Do not Settle for Low-value Partners.</u>

H i Queen, I'm glad to see you here. Now, we are going to be levelling up in our relationship. In this section, I am going to talk about high-value partners and why we don't settle for anything less on our journey to becoming our dream girl. I know some of you ladies are not interested in having a partner, and that is fine. But for the girls who are trying to know what to look for when picking a partner, this section is for you.

Just because they are financially well-to-do doesn't make them a high-value partner. Being financially stable is a good sign, but that isn't the whole pie. Did you know that 51% of first marriages in the U.S.A end in divorce? So, statistically speaking, 1 out of 2 marriages would fail. And 60%-70% of second marriages end in divorce. As THE girl, we don't want to be part of that statistic. So, we are going to be looking at tips for making sure you pick the right one because we don't want to end up 10, 20 years down the line regretting our partner choices.

Below are some tips on how to pick a high-value partner.

Tips on How to Pick a High Value Partner

Shared Values and Goals:

- Look for a partner who shares similar values, beliefs, and long-term goals. Compatibility in fundamental aspects of life can contribute to a stronger and more fulfilling relationship.

Communication Skills:

- Effective communication is crucial in any relationship. A high-value partner is someone who can communicate openly, honestly, and respectfully. Pay attention to how well you understand each other and navigate disagreements.

Respect and Support:

- A high-value partner respects and supports you in your personal and professional endeavors. They celebrate your successes, provide encouragement during challenges, and value your individuality.

Emotional Intelligence:

- Look for a partner with emotional intelligence who understands their own emotions and is empathetic towards yours. Emotional intelligence contributes to better conflict resolution and overall relationship satisfaction.

Trustworthiness:

- Trust is the foundation of a healthy relationship. A high-value partner is trustworthy, reliable, and consistent in their actions.

Trust is built over time through transparency and honesty.

Mutual Growth:

- Seek a partner who encourages personal and mutual growth. A high-value partner is supportive of your aspirations and actively engages in personal development. Together, you both contribute to each other's growth.

Adaptability and Flexibility:

- Life is dynamic, and circumstances change. A high-value partner is adaptable and flexible, able to navigate challenges and changes with resilience and a positive attitude.

Financial Compatibility:

- While money isn't the only factor, it's important to discuss and understand each other's financial values, habits, and goals. Compatibility in financial matters can reduce stress in the relationship.

Shared Interests and Hobbies:

- While differences can be enriching, having shared interests and hobbies can strengthen your bond and provide opportunities for quality time together.

Healthy Boundaries:

- A high-value partner respects healthy boundaries. They understand

the importance of maintaining individual identities and are supportive of your need for personal space and autonomy.

Conflict Resolution Skills:

· Assess how your partner handles conflicts. A high-value partner
communicates constructively, seeks solutions, and doesn't resort
to manipulation or harmful behaviors during disagreements.

Similar Life Priorities:

· Ensure that your partner's life priorities align with yours. This
includes considerations such as family planning, career aspirations,
and lifestyle choices.

Cultural and Religious Compatibility:

· If cultural or religious factors are important to you, consider how
well your values align in these areas. Shared cultural or religious
backgrounds can contribute to a deeper connection.

Physical and Emotional Well-being:

· A high-value partner values and prioritizes both physical and
emotional well-being. They encourage a healthy lifestyle and
prioritize mental health.

Remember that everyone is unique, and there's no one-size-fits-all
formula for choosing a partner. Take the time to get to know the person,
communicate openly, and observe how they handle various aspects of
life. Trust your instincts and prioritize qualities that are important to

you for a fulfilling and lasting relationship.

Alright, so now you know what you want in a partner: the well-off, mature, emotionally intelligent, empathetic partner. The next question is how do you attract such a partner?

Well, I used to say life is a game, and at birth, you are dealt a hand. Some people are dealt really good hands, born to a rich, loving home, built like a god or goddess, and some people not so great. But once you are born, you just have to play the hand life dealt you. Imagine how awesome it would be that you still win at the game of life, no matter the hand life dealt you. Winning in life, to me, is living the best, most fulfilling version of your life. So winning in life might look different for different people, but the goal is to be happy.

I also think, no matter how bad the cards life dealt you are, you will always have that one good card. It might be good health, being smart, looking attractive, born in a good country, etc., but at least, we all have one good card. The trick is to use what you have to get what you want; that's how you win.

So you weren't born rich, but you were born smart; you can use your brain to get money. You weren't born pretty, but you have money; you can use your money to get the beauty you want. The secret is using what you have to get what you want.

Anyhow, back to the task at hand: How to attract a high-value partner. Here are some tips to do that.

How to attract a high value partner

Know Your Worth:

· Understand and appreciate your own value. Confidence in yourself and your worth will naturally attract those who recognize and appreciate it.

Self-Improvement:

- Focus on personal development and self-improvement. Cultivate your interests, talents, and skills. A well-rounded and self-assured individual is often attractive to high-value partners.

Set Clear Boundaries:

- Establish and communicate clear boundaries. A high-value man respects and appreciates individuals who know what they want and can assert their needs.

Be Genuine:

- Be authentic and true to yourself. Authenticity is attractive, and a high-value man is likely to appreciate someone who is genuine and sincere.

Positive Mindset:

- Maintain a positive mindset and outlook on life. Positivity can be contagious and create an attractive energy around you.

Confidence Without Arrogance:

- Project confidence, but avoid arrogance. Confidence is attractive, but humility and the ability to listen are equally important.

Cultivate Your Interests:

- Pursue your passions and interests. Engaging in activities you love not only makes you more interesting but also provides opportunities to meet like-minded individuals.

Effective Communication:

- Develop strong communication skills. Express yourself clearly and actively listen. Communication is vital in any relationship, and being a good communicator can make you more appealing.

Independence:

- Maintain your independence and avoid being overly reliant on a relationship for fulfillment. High-value individuals often appreciate partners who have their own goals and ambitions.

Dress Well and Take Care of Yourself:

- Present yourself in a way that makes you feel confident. Dressing well and taking care of your physical and mental well-being can enhance your attractiveness.

Show Kindness and Empathy:

- Be kind and empathetic. High-value individuals often appreciate those who treat others with respect and compassion.

Be Supportive:

- Be supportive of your partner's goals and aspirations. A high-value man will appreciate a partner who encourages and supports their endeavors.

Cultivate a Positive Lifestyle:

· Create a positive and fulfilling lifestyle. Focus on your own happiness and well-being, and a high-value partner is likely to be drawn to the positive energy you radiate.

Be Open to Love:

· Approach relationships with an open heart. Be willing to connect emotionally and build a genuine connection with the right person.

Remember that attraction is subjective, and what one person values may differ from another. Be patient and stay true to yourself. Building a healthy, lasting connection is often based on mutual respect, shared values, and genuine compatibility.

With a few tips, I'm sure you would be on the path to attracting the type of partner you desire. Also, don't forget to watch out for red flags in the early stages of a relationship; I would absolutely hate for you to end up with a manipulative narcissist.

How to Be a Girl's Girl: Building a community

In a patriarchal society, becoming a girl's girl is a must because we believe in women supporting women. When you are eating healthy and your finances are in order (or getting in order), and you have the partner or pet you want, now you need a support system. As you know, humans are social beings; you need a community.

Making friends when you are younger is easier, but as you grow older, you notice it might be hard to start and maintain meaningful relationships. Well, not to worry, I have some tips to help you with that

Tips on How to Make Girlfriends

Be Approachable:

- Approachability is key to making friends. Smile, make eye contact, and be open to initiating conversations.

Attend Social Events:

- Attend social events, gatherings, or group activities where you can meet new people. This provides a natural context for making connections.

Be Genuine:

- Be yourself and be genuine in your interactions. Authenticity helps build trust and forms the basis for lasting friendships.

Find Common Interests:

- Identify common interests with other women. Whether it's hobbies, sports, or shared values, common ground creates a strong foundation for friendship.

Initiate Conversations:

- Take the initiative to start conversations. Ask open-ended questions and show genuine interest in getting to know others.

Active Listening:

- Practice active listening. Pay attention to what others are saying, and respond thoughtfully. This fosters a sense of connection and understanding.

Join Clubs or Groups:

- Join clubs, groups, or organizations related to your interests. This provides a structured environment for meeting like-minded women.

Offer Support:

- Be supportive and offer help when needed. Building friendships often involves being there for others during both good and challenging times.

Share Personal Experiences:

- Open up about your own experiences, thoughts, and feelings. Vulnerability can deepen connections and create a sense of trust.

Celebrate Achievements:

- Celebrate the achievements and successes of your female friends. This positive reinforcement strengthens the bond between you.

Make Plans:

- Take the initiative to make plans and invite others to join. Whether it's grabbing coffee, attending an event, or having a movie night, making plans fosters a sense of camaraderie.

Respect Differences:

· Respect and appreciate the differences among your friends. Embrace diversity, as it can enrich the dynamics of the friendship.

Be Reliable:

· Be reliable and trustworthy. Being consistent and dependable in your actions helps build a strong foundation for trust.

Apologize and Forgive:

· Inevitably, misunderstandings can occur. Be willing to apologize if needed, and be forgiving when others make mistakes. Healthy friendships involve mutual understanding and forgiveness.

Give Time to Develop:

· Building strong friendships takes time. Be patient and allow relationships to develop naturally over time.

Remember that building friendships is a two-way street. Both parties contribute to the growth and sustainability of the relationship. Be proactive in fostering connections, and prioritize the quality of your interactions over quantity.

Relationships with Family and Loved Ones

When it comes to fostering meaningful connections with family and loved ones, I won't delve too deeply into specifics. The guidebook has surpassed my initial expectations in length, and every family dynamic is uniquely different. You know your family and what works best for you, so trust your instincts. The only advice I would offer is this: if you can nurture positive relationships with your family and loved ones, please do so, as family plays a crucial role, and having a supportive network is invaluable.

5

Conclusion

H ey there, you made it this far, and I'm thrilled that you've journeyed through the guidebook. I hope you've absorbed the tips, tricks, and advice generously sprinkled throughout these pages. If you're still a work in progress, that's perfectly fine. Let's quickly recap what we've covered in the book – the journey to becoming the girl of your dreams. We delved into the three big aspects to get in order: health, finance, and relationships. Armed with the knowledge from this book, I'm confident you can transform into the girl you've always dreamed of being. Consider this book a guiding light on your journey from where you are now to where you want to be. Much love to all. Stay happy, Queens.

If you found this book helpful, I would truly appreciate it if you could leave a favorable review on Amazon.

6

Resources

D*ivorce rate in the U.S.: Geographic Variation, 2022.* (n.d.). Bowling Green State University. https://www.bgsu.edu/ncfmr/resources/data/family-profiles/loo-divorce-rate-US-geographic-variation-2022-fp-23-24.html

Politi, M. (2021, July 25). 28 Millionaire Statistics: What Percentage of Americans Are Millionaires? Linkedin. Retrieved January 28, 2024, from https://www.linkedin.com/pulse/28-millionaire-statistics-what-percentage-americans-politi%3FtrackingId=NkAAW9MuSha7ZaSyQjFcpQ%253D%253D/?trackingId=NkAAW9MuSha7ZaSyQjFcpQ%3D%3D

Author, B. (n.d.). Despite Rising Costs, College Is Still a Good Investment - Liberty Street Economics. Liberty Street Economics. https://libertystreeteconomics.newyorkfed.org/2019/06/despite-rising-costs-college-is-still-a-good-investment/

Printed in Great Britain
by Amazon

38083690R00036